SALT:
Black America's
SILENT KILLER

SALT:
Black America's
SILENT KILLER

Surender Reddy Neravetla, MD, FACS
Director
Cardiac Surgery
Springfield Regional Medical Center

with
Shantanu Reddy Neravetla, MD

Health Now Books, LLC
Springfield, Ohio

Health Now Books, LLC
3484 Rockview Drive
Springfield, Ohio 45504
healthnowbooks.com

ISBN 978-1-938009-04-4 (full-color book)
ISBN 978-1-938009-03-7 (ePub e-book)

For more information about the dangers of
salt consumption and other health-related issues,
please visit healthnowbooks.com.

Acknowledgments

My first thanks go to Sharon Cook, Cook Public Relations, who pointed out the need for this book and persuaded me to undertake this project. Many thanks for her continued encouragement and guidance.

Special thanks go out to the following leaders of the Black American community who helped review the manuscript and provide guidance:

- Rev. Darryl L. Grayson, group coordinator and pastor, Mt. Zion Baptist Church, Springfield, Ohio. Member, board of trustees, Community Mercy Health Partners, Springfield, Ohio.
- Pamela Young, past chairman, board of trustees, Community Mercy Health Partners, Springfield, Ohio. Assistant professor, educational leadership, and director of accreditation, School of Education and Allied Professions, University of Dayton, Dayton, Ohio.
- Germaine Bennett, longtime educator and school administrator. Chair of the board of directors of Mercy Health Partners Southwest Ohio.
- Tara-Nicholle Nelson, Esq., founder, RETHINK Multimedia, San Francisco, California.

Acknowledgments

Thanks to Tina Pavlatos from Visual Anatomy for her translation of my ideas into illustrations and to Jennifer Omner for the cover and book design and layout.

Thanks to Scott Burns, Inspired Media Online, for help with getting out the word on the Web.

Thanks to copy editor Cory Jubitz, of the three c's, for her meticulous attention to detail.

Thanks to many of my family members, my office staff and my coworkers for their continued participation and encouragement.

Finally, thanks once again to my writing coach and editor, Linden Gross, who was instrumental in helping me formulate my ideas and present them in clear and persuasive language.

Contents

Introduction

Black Americans' lives are being cut disgracefully short. More than 40 million Black Americans suffer from health problems that are killing them faster and earlier than their Caucasian counterparts. In a country where the average life expectancy is 78, the average life span of Black Americans is just 70 years. As a result, Black America ranks well below 100 of the world's nations when it comes to longevity.

Given that America has the most expensive and arguably the most technologically advanced health care system in the world, these statistics are very alarming. But we're not just talking about shorter lives. Since life expectancy is a measure of the overall status of a population's health, we're talking about compromised lives as well.

The health problems that cause this lower life expectancy disable many times more people than the actual number killed. Four out of five stroke victims, for example, go on to live for years with severe disabilities. The same holds true for patients with end-stage kidney failure who require dialysis. Strokes and kidney disease are of specific concern to the Black American community since we know that:

- One third of Americans on dialysis are Black Americans. That number is nearly three times higher than one would expect, since Black Americans compose just 13 percent of the country's population.

- Black Americans suffer from significantly higher blood pressure than do their Caucasian counterparts, which, as you are about to see, increases the risk not only of stroke but of a host of other life-threatening health problems as well.

In short, Black Americans experience health problems in a far greater proportion than they should relative to their percentage of the population. We're not just talking about health problems among the elderly. This pattern impacts Black Americans across the age spectrum.

These disturbing facts, often referred to as the "state of Black America," have been attributed to a lack of access to appropriate health care and the related inability of Black Americans to get preventive care or receive early diagnosis and treatment for many known health problems in a timely manner.

As a member of the medical community in the Dayton-Springfield area for nearly three decades, I have often been made aware of the barriers to adequate medical care in certain areas of town. I know from talking to my colleagues from other parts of the country that the same issues exist all over America.

Many economic, social and cultural issues certainly do contribute to higher blood pressure and its consequences among Black Americans. A 2010 report titled "A Closer Look at African American Men and High Blood Pressure Control"[1]

---

1 Centers for Disease Control and Prevention: A Closer Look at African American Men and High Blood Pressure Control: A Review of Psychosocial Factors and Systems-Level Interventions. Atlanta: U.S. Department of Health and Human Services; 2010. www.cdc.gov/bloodpressure/docs/African_American_Executive_Summary.pdf.

commissioned by the Centers for Disease Control and Prevention (CDC) provides a good summary of these socioeconomic and cultural reasons. The following is largely taken from the report of this team consisting of 22 select professionals. The points presented are strongly supported by extensive research data and bibliography:

- Racism:

    The most often quoted and suspected reasons for higher blood pressure and its consequences among Black Americans are real and perceived discrimination and racism.

    Public health researcher and epidemiologist Sherman James coined the term "John Henryism" while investigating racial health disparities to explain the strategy for coping with prolonged exposure to stresses such as social discrimination. Even in this day and age, African Americans, according to many reports, often experience higher stress and perceive discrimination in the workplace. African American workers with higher John Henryism indeed have been found to manifest higher blood pressure.

- Beliefs and attitudes:

    A prevailing attitude of masculinity among many African Americans holds them back from seeking medical care. Preventive care, which by definition requires screening and treatment before any manifestation of symptoms, is met with a perception of inferiority and loss of strength and virility. Masculinity, on the other hand, is defined as independence and strength. Since seeking help is viewed as a sign of weakness, African Americans with this belief are also less likely to access available medical care and accept and follow medical recommendations. Other contributing attitudes and beliefs include a mistrust of the medical establishment and non-African American physicians. As a result, controlling high blood pressure—even after diagnosis—has been difficult.

- Economic status:

  It should come as no surprise to read that African Americans on average are economically disadvantaged compared with White Americans. Lower economic status has been a strong predictor of high blood pressure among Black Americans, much more so than among White Americans of lower economic status. Cultural and economic isolation, lack of insurance, lack of sufficient health care facilities in racially isolated neighborhoods and cost of medications have all been cited as reasons for higher blood pressure and more related complications among African Americans.

The above CDC-sponsored report is one of many sources of such information. This report, like many others, also concludes that even accounting for all of the above psychosocial and socioeconomic factors, African Americans still suffer higher hypertension rates than do White Americans.

As you'll learn in this book, high blood pressure threatens everything from our hearts to our brains to our kidneys. But those are far from the only health challenges that hit Black Americans harder than their Caucasian counterparts. Black Americans are also more likely to suffer from asthma, obesity, stomach cancer and osteoporosis.

Sources of Mortality Differences Between Black and Caucasian Americans

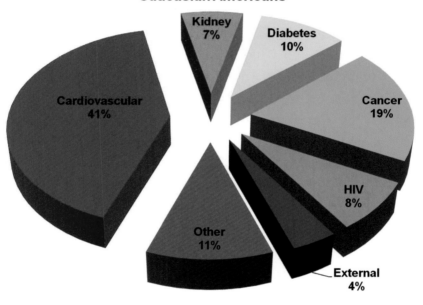

Over the past 200 years, the valiant efforts of many organizations to address the complex social, economic and historical issues leading to Black Americans' dismal state of health have met with only limited success. Despite all the hard work, *largely preventable causes* that lead to heart attacks, strokes and kidney failure account for twice the number of deaths than those from cancers.

Presented in this slender book is an astonishingly simple measure that could help millions of Black Americans. Research reveals that our long-term habit of adding salt to our diet is much more deadly and disabling for Black Americans than for the general population. I will explore the science behind this research specifically as it pertains to Black Americans, along with theories toward the end of the book about why this particular segment of our population is so dreadfully impacted by the overconsumption of salt. My hope is to convince Black Americans to eliminate as much salt as possible from their diets.

People generally don't want to accept the idea that salt is bad for them. They like the taste of salt and can't imagine enjoying food without it. But cutting salt is a lot easier than most people think, especially when reduced gradually. You quickly learn to appreciate the real taste of food when it's not covered up by salt. And you'll definitely appreciate the health benefits now and especially later in life.

Of course, telling people to change their habits to create a better future for themselves generally doesn't work. Over the years, even my closest family members and friends have generally ignored my advice in this regard. All this changed, however, once *Salt Kills* was published. In a few short weeks following its publication, just about anybody who had a chance to read my book dramatically changed his or her habits. The simple language, interesting analogies and creative graphs, all of which are based on a solid foundation of data from medical research, have proven to be very effective. Readers of *Salt Kills* frequently call the book "the Dr. Seuss' *Cat in the Hat*" of health care writing.

This book, *Salt: Black America's Silent Killer*, which uses the same reader-friendly approach, will lead you to a good understanding of how extensively—and in how many differ-ent ways—the salt habit hurts Black Americans. By the end, I hope you realize how the state of Black America's health could be fundamentally improved simply by reducing or eliminat-ing salt consumption. Cutting out salt is such an easy way to dramatically impact Black America's health, especially when compared with other potential solutions. You can call it the low-hanging fruit that's ripe for easy picking. Eliminating salt from a diet does not require huge organization or effort. It sim-ply takes a good understanding of the known facts.

Whether you're an individual seeking better health, a con-cerned parent, a community leader or a health care professional working within the Black American community, this book is for you and all those around you. This one small change could drastically improve the lives and future health of Black Ameri-cans. So please take a careful look at what I have to say. And once you're convinced, I encourage you to join me in spreading the word. Together, we can make Black America healthy.

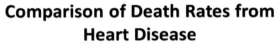

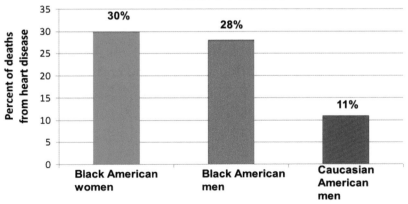

Chapter

1

Salt: The Silent Killer in Your Kitchen

The addition of salt to our daily food, while not healthy for anybody, is downright horrible for Black Americans. Let's explore this problem starting with the following real-life scenario.

The phone rings at three in the morning. The nurse from the ICU apologetically says, "I am sorry to wake you up, Doc. I cannot get the blood pressure of this post-bypass heart surgery patient under control." She goes on. "I know you are worried about bleeding problems after his heart surgery. I have already used the maximum doses of three different medications. I am still not able to bring down the blood pressure."

Take any one of the hundreds of thousands of people who undergo heart bypass operations each year and you will see a vertical scar right in the middle of the chest. During a typical open-heart surgery, the breastbone, which is in the front of the chest, is cut open to allow access to the heart. At the end of the surgery, steel wires are used to bring the two halves of the breastbone together. The new bypasses created during surgery are sewn in place with very fine thread. If the patient's blood pressure rises too high after the operation is concluded and the chest is already closed, the raw cut edges of the bone can start to bleed from the heightened pressure. Any of the delicate suture lines on the heart could also break from the same high pressure, causing bleeding.

This bleeding is dangerous because the blood will accumulate around the heart and prevent the heart from pumping well. If a suture line snaps from this high pressure, the sudden loss of a lot of blood could be disastrous. So you can understand why the nurse taking care of this patient is worried. I give orders to switch to a stronger class of medication and higher doses. I hope the pressure comes down, because there's nothing more that I—or anyone else—can do.

This conversation highlights the problem Black Americans face in dealing with salt-induced high blood pressure. Our bodies are made up of water in which a variety of different kinds of salts, called electrolytes, have been dissolved. The concentration of these electrolytes—or salts—in the body is maintained with scrupulous precision by complex mechanisms. What happens when that balance is thrown off, say by our eating excess salt? If the fluid around the blood cells has too high a concentration of salt, our blood cells will release some of their fluid into the surrounding fluid. Balance is restored, but at a cost, because the cells that have provided the necessary fluid wind up dying since they no longer have enough fluid to stay healthy. Conversely, if the salt concentration in each cell is higher than that of the surrounding fluid, the fluid will permeate the cells to even things out. The extra fluid causes the cells to swell like balloons and, eventually, like balloons that get overfilled, to burst.

As you can see, adding extra salt to your food causes direct damage on the cellular level. Of course, our bodies do have additional resources to help with the salt overload—namely our kidneys. By controlling the composition of our urine, the kidneys can help maintain the right balance of electrolytes to a point. Over time, however, they just can't handle all the excess salt we consume. So the kidneys also cause us to retain water in order to balance out the fluids in and around the blood cells.

When you retain water, the pressure in the blood vessels goes up due to the higher volume of fluids in your body. It's as simple as that. If you have any doubt about this salt and water connection, just try eating salty potato chips or peanuts; you will pretty much be forced to drink some liquids. If you then drink a soda pop instead of a glass of water, the food-processing and beverage industries have it made, especially since sodas contain salt. You'll want to continue eating your salty snack and drinking your salty soda. Why else do you think that these industries fight any salt restriction in processed foods?

These industries are profiting at the expense of your physical well-being. You probably know the feeling that comes with retaining water. Suddenly it's hard to slip on your rings or even your shoes. That's because the volume of water that your system now has to deal with has increased, but the system of blood vessels through which this water circulates has not.

What happens when you stuff a suitcase so full that you

have to sit on it to get it closed? More often than not, the zipper pops. It just can't hold up against all that pressure.

Your body works the same way. All that extra pressure—in this case, blood pressure—that results from having to compensate for an excess of salt in your system eventually wreaks havoc on your body, causing it to malfunction in a number of ways. That's especially true for Black Americans.

Eating salty processed foods or adding salt in home cooking causes Black Americans to suffer high blood pressure and many other consequences at a much greater rate and often with greater intensity than White Americans. That's because, as I will explain at greater length in this book, Black Americans are more sensitive to salt than are Caucasian Americans. This salt sensitivity is largely responsible for Black America's poor state of health and the main reason for Black American life expectancy ranking below that of 100 of the world's nations.

Data gathered from prominent sources such as the American Heart Association reveal that:

- Black Americans have high blood pressure almost twice as often as Caucasian Americans.
- Severe high blood pressure, which is greater than 180 mm Hg, is encountered almost six times more often in African Americans with high blood pressure than in Caucasian Americans.
- This high blood pressure, just as with the heart patient I wrote about at the beginning of this chapter, is much more difficult to control. Stronger medications, higher doses and combinations of medications are usually needed, but they do not always work to lower dangerous blood pressure levels.

- Black Americans have high blood pressure at an earlier age.
- The degree of the problem is also higher, meaning that Black Americans suffer a higher rate of complications from a similar degree of high blood pressure than do White Americans.
- The target organ damage to the heart, kidney and brain from high blood pressure is disproportionately greater.
- Among Black Americans, the risk of high blood pressure goes up even more with obesity, inactivity and diabetes, all of which are also unfortunately more common compared with Caucasian Americans.

Salt-related health problems don't stop with high blood pressure. As I mentioned earlier, Black Americans pay a much higher penalty with salt-related health problems, including asthma, stomach cancer, osteoporosis, obesity and dementia.

Why such a vast difference?

The answer lies in the fact that Black Americans are very sensitive to salt intake.

Chapter

Salt Sensitivity

If your blood pressure does not go up when challenged with a salt-loaded meal, you are called *salt resistant*. If your blood pressure does go up, then you are *salt sensitive*.

The idea of salt sensitivity goes way back to 1950, when researcher Dr. R.B. Maneely and co-researchers conducted experiments on rats showing that the average blood pressure of a rat went up in proportion to the salt added to the rat's diet. Other researchers showed the same pattern in several different animals, including chimpanzees, which have the closest genetic match to humans.

This groundbreaking research also revealed that while the rats as a group responded to salt with high blood pressure, there was a marked degree of individual variation. So Dr. Lewis K. Dahl began investigating the difference in the response to salt among rats. He worked for decades at the Brookhaven National Laboratory in Upton, New York, a highly regarded lab that has made many contributions to present-day medical care. Dr. Dahl and his co-researchers were able to separate the rats into two groups based on their response to salt—whether they were sensitive or resistant. After a period of inbreeding, he then created two distinctive lines of rats: salt-sensitive S rats and salt-resistant R rats.

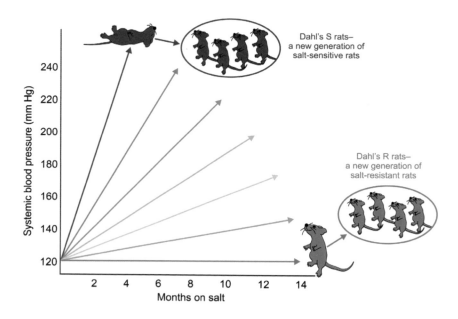

The awareness of salt sensitivity among animal models has led to the study of various ethnic groups to determine how they respond to a salt challenge. Whereas only 25 percent of White Americans are salt sensitive, nearly two thirds of Black Americans are salt sensitive. Not surprisingly, nearly all (95 percent of) salt-sensitive Black Americans go on to have high blood pressure. So there is a direct link between the common prevalence of high blood pressure and salt sensitivity.

Pervasive salt-induced high blood pressure among Black

Americans is taking its toll. Nearly three quarters of the difference in life expectancy between Black and White Americans comes from premature deaths caused by salt-induced and salt-sensitive high blood pressure. Put another way, salt-induced high blood pressure causes the death of nearly one out of every two Black Americans.

As we saw in the Introduction, the premature deaths of Black Americans from salt-induced high blood pressure does not take into account the number of people living with disabilities and dysfunctions caused by the same problem. Millions of Black Americans live with stroke, kidney failure and more (which we'll be discussing), all as a result of salt-induced high blood pressure. In view of this disproportionally severe high blood pressure caused by habitual salt intake among the Black American population, it should come as no surprise that Black Americans also suffer from a variety of heart problems due to salt sensitivity.

Salt Sensitivity and Survival

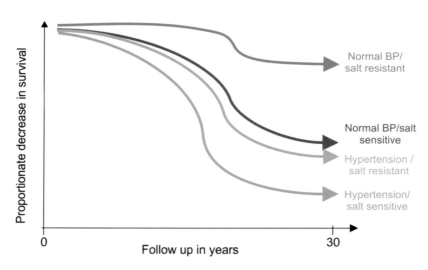

Chapter

The Heart

Heart attacks are twice as prevalent among Black Americans as they are among Caucasian Americans. And that's just the start when it comes to the heart problems suffered by Black Americans.

Why do heart problems affect the Black American community so disproportionately?

It starts with high blood pressure, which over time takes a relatively straight artery and begins to twist it. We're not just talking about small kinks. High blood pressure can actually cause the artery to bend on itself like a hairpin turn on a winding road. As a result, the blood that once flowed freely through unobstructed arteries is now getting bounced off the artery walls at every turn. And since it's flowing with high pressure (that's what high blood pressure means), eventually the repeated pounding of the blood against those curvy parts of the artery walls does damage to the inside lining of the arteries.

Normal Blood Pressure   High Blood Pressure

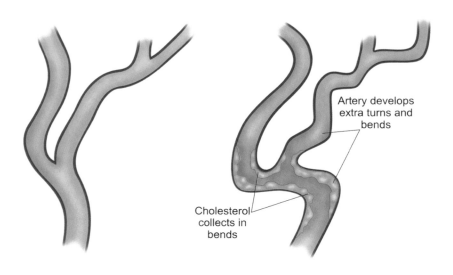

Artery develops
extra turns and
bends

Cholesterol
collects in
bends

Those indents along our artery walls are like shallow caves that cholesterol deposits soon wind up calling home. Eventually those cholesterol deposits grow large enough to block the flow of blood. And while procedures exist to clear clogged arteries with wires and catheters, it's almost impossible to "roto-rooter" a crooked artery.

That explains why cardiovascular disease related to cholesterol (or fat) deposits in our arteries and blood vessels is by far the largest killer of people around the world. When the heart no longer receives its blood supply because the artery that delivers the blood has gotten blocked by cholesterol deposits, you suffer a heart attack. A portion of your heart literally dies.

Cholesterol buildup (often caused by salt-induced high blood pressure) can also weaken the wall of the aorta, the large artery that originates from the heart, causing a bulge known as an aneurysm. If the aneurysm gets large enough, it ruptures, allowing all the blood inside the arterial system to escape. Death follows rather quickly.

Differences in Hypertension Rates

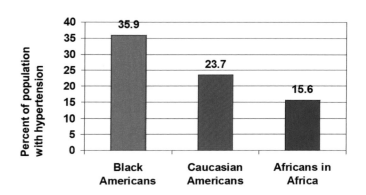

Percentages of Hypertensive Americans with Severe Hypertension (BP > 180 mm Hg)

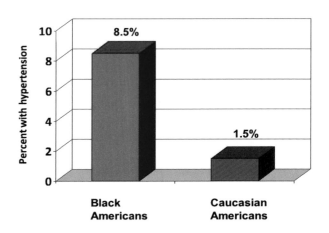

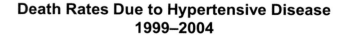

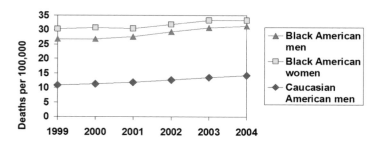

Add up the people who die annually due to all the different kinds of cancers and the total will still be fewer than the number of people who fall victim each year to cardiovascular disease. Salt-induced high blood pressure doubles the risk of an average person falling victim to this mega-killer. Since *salt-sensitive* Black Americans are three times more prone to high blood pressure, their risk of suffering a heart attack is six times greater than White Americans'.

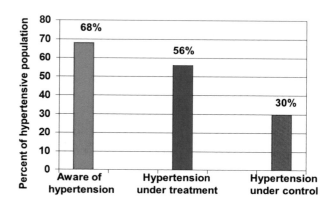

Hypertension in Black Americans

- **Hypertension at an earlier age**
- **Higher blood pressure**
- **More difficult to control**
- More complications

Complications of Hypertension in Black Americans

- **Death from stroke increased four times**
- Heart disease **increased three times**
- **Heart failure risk doubled**
- Renal failure **increased three times**

To make matters worse, the lucky few Black Americans who are not sensitive also pay an extraordinarily heavy price for their salt habit. Individuals who don't have high blood pressure can still experience hardening of the arteries in response to salt intake.

Whether you have high blood pressure or hardening of the arteries, the impact on the heart is much the same—it has to work harder to pump the blood through your body. If you go to a gym and work any one group of muscles against resistance for about 20 minutes at a time and only twice a week, that group of muscles will grow bigger. Biceps curls would be a good example of this. When you have salt-induced high blood pressure, your poor heart is having a workout 24/7 with each and every heartbeat. The heart muscle grows just like any other muscle. So high blood pressure naturally creates a big heart.

You might think having a big heart is a good thing. Think again.

The Big Heart

I was in Atlanta in spring 2012 attending a conference. That trip brought into focus for me the dire need to alert Black Americans to the dangers of habitual salt intake.

We went to watch an Atlanta Braves baseball game in Turner Field. One of the locals in our party said, "You should try some boiled peanuts." He loves them so much that he brags that "boiled peanuts are the specialty of Turner Field. They taste so good—these peanuts are to die for."

With an introduction like that, we had to try these boiled peanuts. And so we did.

My goodness, they were so intolerably salty that I spit out the very first boiled peanut I put in my mouth. After a while, I tried another one. Same taste. I could not handle eating these peanuts at all. I don't remember ever eating something so salty. These peanuts were the closest thing I've experienced to eating plain salt.

Keep in mind that, according to the 2010 Census report, more than half of Atlanta's citizens are Black Americans.

Out of curiosity, I went to have a conversation with the young lady who had sold me the peanuts. She was a sophomore at a local college and worked at the food stand on weekends to help pay for school. Hoping that these peanuts were cooked on site, I asked her if I could get some salt-free boiled peanuts. No such luck. Instead, this young Black American student retorted, "What's wrong with these peanuts? They are a hot seller at Turner Field." After further conversation, it was abundantly clear that she had never heard that adding salt was not good for anybody's health. She had certainly not heard that the implications of adding salt to food are horrendously worse for Black Americans.

As I returned to watch the game, I was thinking about a way to illustrate what happens to the heart when dealing with salt-induced high blood pressure. It occurred to me that baseball is a perfect way to explain this problem, since way back during my medical training we used to call an enlarged heart a *baseball heart*.

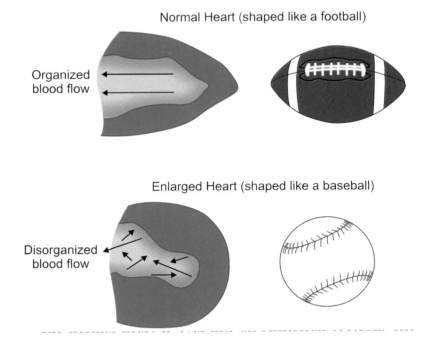

Normal Heart (shaped like a football)

Organized blood flow

Enlarged Heart (shaped like a baseball)

Disorganized blood flow

football-shaped heart has an open end and is closed at the other end. When the walls of the football come together, the contents are forced out from the open end. The forces inside a baseball, on the other hand, are fighting each other, so they cannot pump blood as efficiently. More important, the baseball heart is very rigid and unyielding. I remember conversations with my cardiology colleagues. "Hey, buddy, you told me this was going to be straightforward surgery with a nice, vigorous pumping heart," I've said more than once. "Instead, we found a baseball that was as stiff as a rock with low function."

The baseball heart does manage to pump fairly well. The problem lies in its inability to relax, a much-needed phase of the pumping cycle when the chamber of the heart actually fills with blood. The squeezing part of the pumping cycle, called *systole*, may not be compromised in a big baseball heart. The big heart, however, has difficulty with its relaxing phase, or the *diastole*. The consequences of this are often devastating.

My Heart Is Failing

In just the last five years, we have come to realize that diastolic dysfunction is a major reason why millions of Americans suffer heart failure. To understand diastolic dysfunction and its connection to heart failure, we need to get back to the ball game we were watching.

Halfway through the close ball game, there was a runner on first base. To get the runner in scoring position and onto second base, the manager asked the next batter to bunt. The batter held his bat at knee level and pushed the ball on contact. The ball then traveled only within the infield, giving the first-base runner just enough time to run to second base. Normally, the batter takes his bat all the way back behind his shoulders and then swings through the ball, making contact at knee to thigh level. You can call this phase of the batter's action—when he takes the bat back before swinging it forward—the backswing or the windup. If the batter makes good contact with the ball while swinging forward from the windup, the ball can leave the ballpark for a home run. Indeed, you can hit a home run only when you take a full backswing or a full windup. When you just bunt, the ball can travel only a short distance. So taking a full backswing or windup is a critical part of the batter's swing if the ball is to travel far.

Pastor Darryl Grayson, one of the advisers on this project, pointed out to me that the batter's windup in baseball is also known as "loading." In medicine, we use a similar term with reference to heart function. For instance, filling the heart chamber—thereby stretching the heart muscle—increases the cardiac output much the same way as the batter's windup. We refer to this as the "pre-load," as in loading before pumping. Increasing the pre-load of the heart will increase the output of the heart much the same way that a fully loaded bat swing makes the ball go farther. A solid pre-load gives the heart the power to pump or the baseball the power to sail over the fence. That's where loading stops as far as baseball is concerned. With hearts, however, there's also an "after-load," when blood pressure offers resistance to the pumping action of the heart. The higher the blood pressure—or after-load—the tougher it is for the heart to pump.

A heart muscle constantly having to pump against higher blood pressure caused by the lifelong addition of salt to our food means a heart muscle that's constantly fighting a higher after-load. The result of all that work is that the heart muscle keeps getting bigger and bigger, until it's thick and stiff (and even shaped) like a baseball. Unfortunately, as we have discussed, the baseball heart cannot relax as it used to during the pre-load phase. So a baseball heart increasingly loses its windup or the ability to fully load to the point that it can no longer pump out the blood efficiently. This change takes place slowly and is so subtle that

Normal Heart Muscle

Enlarged Heart Muscle

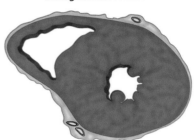

it is usually overlooked. You may simply say to yourself, "I am not a spring chicken anymore. I cannot do the same things I used to before." Or you may notice getting tired easily. While these changes don't seem significant, they are often the earliest signs of heart failure.

When the heart is not able to keep up with the demands placed on it by your activities, we in medicine call it *heart failure*. As your windup continues to be compromised, you will reach a point when your heart is only bunting. Now you are in full-blown heart failure. At this stage, you can barely move around, you are very short of breath and your legs are swollen.

Hospitals in America are filled with people suffering from some type of heart failure, which is the number-one reason for hospitalization for people over 65 years of age. The majority of disabling heart problems and frequent hospitalizations can be traced back to the simple phenomenon of developing a big heart in response to high blood pressure.

Once again, the Black community takes a battering on this front, because Black Americans' hearts are overgrown three times as often as White Americans' hearts. As a result, Black Americans experience sudden cardiac death (you suddenly die even though you've never had any symptoms of heart problems) three times as commonly as do White Americans.

Heart failure not only hits Black Americans more often than it does Caucasian Americans, it hits at a younger age. Finding an overgrown, enlarged heart is common in the Black American population, so much so that in my decades of heart surgery experience I have never seen a heart of a Black American patient—no matter how young—that is not enlarged. The main culprit: habitual intake of salt that causes more severe high blood pressure at a much younger age.

As we've seen, the data show that almost one out of two Black Americans has high blood pressure. You are diagnosed with high blood pressure if it is at or above 140/90 mm Hg. However, if you include those who have blood pressure below 140/90 mm Hg but above 120/80 (pre-hypertension), you will get a better idea of the prevalence of high blood pressure in the Black community and the reason why so many suffer from enlarged hearts. Even a heart muscle fighting pre-hypertension will continue to grow because it's fighting against higher than normal blood pressure.

Clearly, high blood pressure can be deadly. Yet only half of the Black Americans who have high blood pressure are aware of their condition. And only half of those actually get it under control. If you use the pre-hypertension guidelines, the picture gets much worse. In one report, Black Americans below the age of 50 are 20 times more likely to suffer heart failure than are Caucasian Americans.[2] This statistic alone should drive you to stop adding salt to your food so that you don't have to live disabled and dysfunctional with heart failure. Even if you've been fortunate enough to not suffer any other problem with your salt habit, heart failure is almost definitely in your future if you're a salt-using Black American.

Heart trouble among Black Americans is distressing, but that's just the beginning when it comes to salt-induced health problems that are decimating the Black community. Other problems are equally or even more devastating. The heart-breaking penalty Black America pays for kidney failure due to habitual salt intake, for example, makes that by far the most compelling and urgent reason to avoid salt.

---

2   Bibbins-Domingo K, Pletcher MJ, Lin F, Vittinghoff E, Gardin JM, Arynchyn A, Lewis CE, Williams OD, Hulley SB. Racial Differences in Incident Heart Failure Among Young Adults. *New England Journal of Medicine.* 2009 Mar 19;360(12):1179–90. doi: 10.1056/NEJMoa0807265. http://www.ncbi.nlm.nih.gov/pubmed/?term=heart+failure+African+2009+nejm.

Chapter

Renal Failure

High blood pressure triggered by eating salt causes Black Americans to lose kidney function more than four times more commonly than it does for Caucasian Americans. In some pockets of the country, such as the southeastern region, Black Americans' kidney failure has been reported as high as 20 times that of Caucasian Americans.

The medical literature often describes high blood pressure among Black Americans as *clinically severe and biochemically aggressive*. The best evidence of this is that Black Americans suffer kidney damage at a much younger age and in a much higher proportion than any other ethnic group. The kidney, as you have learned, is one of the main target organs to suffer from salt-induced, long-term high blood pressure (the heart and the brain being the other two).

Once the kidneys fail, dialysis is the only way to keep you alive. In dialysis clinics across America, people are hooked up to these machines every other day for up to six hours at a time. What a way to stay alive. I have been called to check on patients in dialysis units many times. I've often been struck by how many Black American patients I see tethered to these machines. From this view, you wouldn't know that Black Americans account for only 13 percent of the U.S. population. It is horrifying that one third of all dialysis patients across America are Black Americans.

In addition to spending a large part of their day in dialysis clinics as well as going in and out of hospitals, patients on dialysis are almost always anemic. So most of the time they don't have nearly enough energy to lead what we consider a normal life. Imagine how that would impact you. Afflicted young Black Americans will have to contend with that limited and disabled life for years to come.

The families of these young Black Americans on dialysis also suffer. One day, I was called to see a patient who needed

Kidney Failure by the Numbers

- **Of the 398,861 American adults on dialysis in 2009, nearly 40% were Black Americans.**
- **90,000 people are currently on a waiting list for a kidney transplant.**
- **Black Americans are 10 years younger than the average patient at the time of their first dialysis.**
- Mean survival for all who start dialysis is only three years.

surgery in order to go on dialysis. This 30-year-old Black American woman had been on dialysis since the birth of her last child. She was diagnosed with very high blood pressure when she was only 20 years of age, and the kidneys had finally quit working during her last pregnancy. Her two children were at her bedside. It was heartbreaking to think of a young mother spending every other day attached to a machine and how that would compromise her ability to attend to her children—or to her own life.

This scenario has played out many times in my career. Compared with Caucasian Americans, Black Americans end up on dialysis at a much younger age. We may accept elderly people having health problems and disabilities, but as in the case of the youthful mother of two, young Black Americans are often robbed of their productive lives by kidney failure.

The story of our Black mother of two gets even worse. Like all dialysis patients, she needed surgery that would allow the

Relative Probability of Being Placed on Dialysis

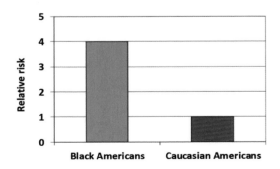

Black Americans are four times more likely to suffer from end-stage kidney failure leading to dialysis.

dialysis machine to be attached. This surgical procedure, called a *shunt*, creates a large connection between an artery and a vein that can be accessed by the dialysis machine. Unfortunately, after functioning for a period of time, these shunts often fail. A young person such as this woman could end up with repeated operations starting from one wrist to the forearm to the other side and then going to the upper arms. Eventually you have to start all over again at the initial shunt's site. In short, since the shunts only last for a limited time in most people, it's a never-ending, frustrating and painful cycle of surgeries.

The experience of taking care of these types of patients proved so disheartening to me that I could no longer stomach it, especially after my wife and I had our first child. I just could not bear to see so many young people (most of whom were Black American) hooked up to those dialysis machines. Since then, I have developed a healthy respect for the physicians who specialize in—and continue to deliver care for—people in kidney failure.

Getting a kidney transplant would be a way out of this misery for many. However, Black Americans on the waiting list for organ donation are up to 75 percent less likely than Caucasian Americans to get an organ transplant. While waiting for donor kidneys, an estimated 150,000 Black Americans (more than a third of the 398,861 patients on dialysis) fill dialysis centers across the United States.

The dismal picture gets even worse. Once placed on dialysis, the life expectancy of young Black Americans is very low. Despite modern medical technology, a 40-year-old without functioning kidneys may not live even eight years. Compare that with an average American, who at age 49 is still expected to live another 33 years. Life expectancy is further reduced in Black Americans on dialysis who also have diabetes as well as in—get this—those who continue to add salt to their food.

The severe elevation of blood pressure in response to habitual salt intake is at the center of this grotesque problem of kidney failure. Young Black Americans do not have to pay this severe cost of compromised lives and premature deaths from kidney failure. Their unnecessary suffering could be prevented simply by not adding salt to their diets.

Unfortunately, there's a lot more bad news related to salt and Black Americans. The next target of the wrath of habitual salt intake is the brain.

Chapter

Stroke

The Black American population is affected by stroke more than any other group. Similar to kidney failure, more Black Americans at a younger age suffer strokes from clinically aggressive, salt-induced high blood pressure. The rate of stroke is double that of Caucasian Americans, and Black American stroke sufferers are twice as likely to die from strokes. The ones who survive are more apt to become disabled and experience difficulties with daily living and activities.

Stroke victims can be so challenged that they often tell you they are "living a life worse than death." Just picture this: If you suffer a stroke to the left side of the brain, you will not be able to talk or use the right side of the body. You will not be able to use your right hand to feed yourself or use your right leg to stand, much less walk. You will need assistance to attend to the most basic needs of the body, such as feeding, bathing and going to the bathroom. And all while you are fully awake, alert and aware of what is happening to you. No wonder stroke victims and their families often say, "You do not wish this on your worst enemy."

Each year nearly 800,000 Americans—a third of them Black Americans—suffer a stroke. Loss of blood flow to a part of the brain is the most common cause of strokes. High blood pressure increases the risk of cholesterol buildup in the arteries that carry blood to the brain. From time to time, this cholesterol plaque completely blocks the blood flow or breaks loose

Carotid Surgery

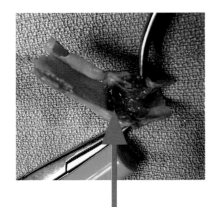

Cholesterol in the artery in the neck.

Cholesterol from the same artery. Note the irregular surface, ulceration and clot.

and blocks an artery farther down. In either event, the part of the brain that was getting the blood flow from that particular artery dies.

High blood pressure, a severe degree of which is much more common among Black Americans, can also cause a stroke when a small artery in the brain ruptures due to the pressure. Blood suddenly exits the arterial system and intrudes into the tissues of the brain. Part of the brain dies from a loss of blood supply. Even more of the brain around the initial area of stroke dies due to the pressure built up from the escaped blood and clot contained within the enclosed, limited space of the skull.

High blood pressure has a drastic and direct correlation to your likelihood of suffering a stroke. At a systolic blood pressure of 180 mm Hg (the top number of your blood pressure), the stroke risk is eight times greater than at 120 mm Hg. We have also learned that not all medications commonly used to treat high blood pressure make it into the arteries of the brain. Blood pressure readings show the blood pressure in your arm, not your brain. So you could therefore be under the impression that the high blood pressure is under control as measured by the cuff around your arm and yet still have high blood pressure in the arteries of your brain.

Knowing someone living with a stroke, or simply being able to picture a stroke victim, should convince you to do whatever it takes to avoid such a fate. Cutting salt in your diet is such a simple step to take to prevent high blood pressure and one of its collateral damages, the stroke. In the process, you'll be protecting yourself against yet another salt-related threat to your brain.

That's right. As if the risk of suffering a stroke weren't bad enough, eating salt impacts the brain in other ways. Loss of memory is a more subtle yet common consequence of salt-induced high blood pressure.

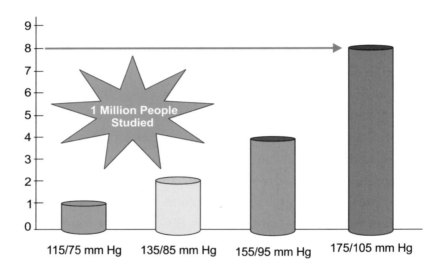

Cardiovascular Mortality and Stroke Risk Doubles for Each 20/10 mm Hg Increase in BP

Chapter

Memory Loss

The Alzheimer's Society reports that having high blood pressure raises the risk of some types of memory loss by six times. That's 600 percent. Not surprisingly, Black Americans, given their predisposition to severe high blood pressure, are almost twice as likely to suffer memory loss.

The statistics are so staggering that health authorities are calling memory loss the fastest-growing health problem in America. The Alzheimer's Society calls it "the silent epidemic." Nearly 50 percent of hospital patients have a clinical diagnosis of dementia, and nearly 85 percent of patients over 50 are estimated to suffer from some form of dementia, including Alzheimer's disease.

You've probably heard of a CAT scan. Not too long ago, a CAT scan was an expensive test, done only in rare circumstances. Nowadays CAT scans of just about any part of the body are routinely performed, almost as frequently as a chest x-ray was done in the past. Going a step further in technology, the MRI is a newer test that's often performed, especially when evaluating the brain and the joints. Both the CAT scan and MRI are frequently used all across America to diagnose diseases of the brain such as tumors, bleeding and strokes.

During these tests, radiologists have commonly found minute scars in different parts of the brain. At first, the significance of these scars was not clear. The radiologists reported them as "age-related" changes in the brain, because the older you are, the more scars you have. For a long time, this finding received no special attention. Having scars in the brain was brushed off by patients the same way that the early signs of heart failure have been dismissed. "Oh, I am not a spring chicken anymore," the afflicted individual reasons. "So I cannot do the same things I used to do a year ago."

Research focused on tracking the health of people with these scars, however, has indicated very serious implications: The more of these so-called age-related scars you have in the brain, the more likely you are to develop memory dysfunction.

This, again, connects back to habitual salt intake, since the higher your blood pressure, the greater the number of scars in your brain (which eventually lead to memory loss). Let me explain why. The gray matter of the brain stores your memory. Scars in the gray matter wipe out the stored memory. Scars in the white matter also impede memory. The white matter of the brain, which is packed with conduction systems, connects with gray matter to recall the stored memory. Scars in the white matter caused by the shearing forces of high blood pressure fracture the brain's electric wiring, so to speak. As a result, you lose the ability to recall the stored memory. Either way, you develop dementia (memory loss).

In 2012, the Alzheimer's Society sounded the alarm bell stating that there is a six-fold increase (not a 6 percent but rather a 600 percent increase) in memory dysfunction with high blood pressure. We know that Black Americans suffer from higher blood pressure more often and to a more severe degree. As a result, Black Americans suffer from memory loss at least twice as often as Caucasian Americans do.

Did You Know?

Nearly 50% of hospital patients have a
clinical diagnosis of dementia.
It is estimated that nearly 85% of patients over 50 suffer
from some form of dementia, including Alzheimer's disease.

The Alzheimer's Association
& The Alois Alzheimer Foundation

Hopefully the notion of avoiding the loss of mental function on top of previously mentioned physical dysfunctions caused by salt-induced illnesses provides enough motivation to cut salt in your diet right now. But the salt-related damage, as bad as it has already been portrayed, doesn't stop here. Hold on, as from the brain, we move to the lungs and the fact that a simple reduction in salt intake could literally mean life and breath for so many Black American children.

Chapter

Asthma

The number of acute asthmatic attacks is directly proportional to salt intake. This is simply due to the retention of excess fluid to compensate for the salt we keep adding to our food. The excess fluid chokes the breathing passages. Once again, Black Americans suffer more frequently on this front, with their children showing up in emergency rooms gasping for breath in a state of acute asthmatic attack four and a half times more often than Caucasian American children.

On top of this unnecessary suffering, Black American children are less likely to survive a seemingly simple asthmatic attack. As a parent myself, it is heartbreaking to say the least to see Black American children suffer death rates from asthma upward of seven times (700 percent) those of Caucasian American children.

Four and a half million Black Americans—mostly children under the age of 18—suffer from asthma. Similar to many

Asthma by the Numbers

- In 2010, almost 4,500,000 non-Hispanic Black Americans had asthma.
- **Black Americans in 2010 were 30% more likely to have asthma than were Caucasian Americans.**
- **In 2009, Black Americans were three times more likely to die from asthma-related causes than were Caucasian Americans.**
- Black American children have death rates seven times those of Caucasian American children.
- Asthma-related emergency room visits are four and a half times more frequent for Black Americans than for Caucasian Americans.

other preventable illnesses related to salt intake, Black Americans are at least 30 percent more likely to suffer asthma than their Caucasian counterparts. Once afflicted by asthma, the Black American child is many times more likely to experience severe difficulty in breathing before potentially dying.

The Proportional Impact of Asthma Prevalence, Health Care Use and Mortality Among Children 0–17 Years of Age, by Race and Ethnicity, United States, 2003–2004			
	Non-Hispanic Black	Non-Hispanic White	Non-Hispanic Black/Non-Hispanic White Ratio
Current prevalence (2004–2005)	146%	92%	1.6
Emergency department visit rate	254%	66%	3.8
Death rate	354%	50%	7.1

Source: CDC 2006. The State of Childhood Asthma, United States, 1980–2005.

Any parent will tell you that it is harder to see your child suffer than yourself. But when suffering and absurdly premature loss of life come from preventable causes, it's simply inexcusable. Think about it. All you have to do to protect your children is to cut back on—or eliminate—their salt consumption.

While you're at it, you might as well cut back on your own. Just in case you need more convincing, here's one more argument. Salt even puts Black Americans at increased risk for stomach cancer, one of the ugliest cancers and most dreadful ways to end one's life.

Chapter

Stomach Cancer

When it comes to cancers, the overall risk of developing any cancer for Black Americans is about the same as it is for Caucasian Americans. However, if you're a Black American, your risk of developing stomach cancer is more than twice that of a Caucasian American. Unfortunately, because of the simple connection between salt and stomach cancer, the Black American population once again pays a disproportionately higher penalty for habitual salt intake.

The most common variety of stomach cancer develops from repeated injury to its inside lining (mucosa). Keep on adding salt to your food, and the initially small areas of damage become larger, turning into what is commonly referred to as stomach ulcers. As you continue to pour salt into these open wounds, some of the ulcers develop into cancers. We still don't know exactly why Black Americans are more predisposed to these cancerous growths in the stomach lining; however, we do know for a fact that they are doubly susceptible.

Cancer is scary. You don't want to have any kind of cancer, but stomach cancer is one of the worst. There has hardly been any progress in the outcome of patients who present with stomach cancer. For starters, the disease grows so imperceptibly that in 90 percent of all cases by the time it's finally detected this cancer has already spread beyond a possible cure. Because of its very low cure rates, stomach cancer remains the second-leading cause of cancer deaths in the world.

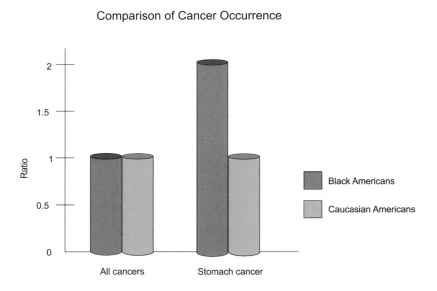

Comparison of Cancer Occurrence

Living with stomach cancer is just horrific. As the cancer continues to grow, you will be able to eat less and less. I don't know if you can imagine a state of living in which you cannot even swallow your own saliva. Not a good way to live or die.

Stomach Cancer

New Cancer Cases per 100,000 Men

Cancer	Black American Men	Caucasian Men	Black American/ Caucasian Ratio
All sites	611.1	540.4	1.1
Colon and rectum	63.3	50	1.3
Lung	92.9	68.4	1.4
Pancreas	18.5	13.8	1.3
Prostate	227.7	147.6	1.5
Stomach	16.3	8.1	2

Source: CDC, 2012

New Cancer Cases per 100,000 Women

Cancer	Black American Women	Caucasian Women	Black American/ Caucasian Ratio
All sites	394.8	437.2	0.9
Breast	122.4	134.8	0.9
Cervical	8.9	6.2	1.4
Colon and rectum	47.6	39.3	1.2
Pancreas	14.9	10.5	1.4
Stomach	7.9	3.6	2.2

Source: CDC, 2012

The Black American population doesn't have to pay this excessive price. Reducing the risk of getting this deadly and disabling cancer should be one of the strongest reasons to cut salt intake. Obesity, and all the other related health complications salt causes, is another.

Chapter

Obesity

I was making the rounds one day when Brenda (not her real name), one of the staff members of the hospital, stopped me in the hallway to share this news. "Guess what, Dr. Neravetla?" she started with excitement in her eyes. "My daughter lost 30 pounds in just a few weeks when she stopped using salt in her food. She has been trying to lose weight without any success for a long time."

I was pleasantly surprised. Quite frankly, when I first started talking to my patients, friends and family members about the need for salt reduction, I was largely focusing on the direct impact of salt-induced high blood pressure on the heart. Since then, I've heard from any number of people who started cutting salt in their food that they were losing unwanted pounds without any other direct effort. In fact, weight reduction has been the most common feedback I have received from people who have cut salt in their diets. As I looked into this further, it became obvious to me that the reduction of salt intake will have a major impact on obesity and the multitude of resulting health problems.

If you look around, it should come as no surprise to learn that we have a problem with obesity in America. By various estimates, one in three Americans is overweight and one in five meets the more strict criteria of obesity. When it comes to Black Americans, we have a bigger problem. One in three Black Americans is obese and almost half are overweight. Black American women are by far the worst affected. More than 80 percent of Black American women are overweight. Consequently, Black Americans are confronted with the damaging effects of being overweight more frequently and more intensely than are Caucasian Americans.

Tackling obesity is perhaps the most far-reaching reason to reduce salt intake, especially for Black Americans. The CDC and other health agencies estimate that more than 300,000 deaths in America can be attributed to obesity annually. According to the National Institutes of Health, obesity and excess weight together are the second-leading cause of preventable death in the United States, close behind tobacco use. A substantial reason for the lower life expectancy of Black Americans is obesity. In addition, countless Black Americans are living with disabilities and dysfunctions caused by obesity.

Not only are lives often prematurely lost, the cost of caring for the multitude of obesity-related illnesses is staggering. The total cost of overweight and obesity to the U.S. economy in 1995 dollars was $99.2 billion—approximately $51.6 billion in direct costs and $47.6 billion in indirect costs.

There are, of course, numerous reasons for this obesity epidemic in the Black American community. We already know that Black Americans do not get the same health care as Caucasian Americans for a variety of socioeconomic and cultural reasons. While there has been little progress in overcoming these challenges over the last many decades, with some education, overcoming the salt habit could prove an easier task and help Black Americans to lose the pounds that are cutting so many lives short and compromising so many others.

The salt and obesity connection is not just my observation. The INTERSALT study,[3] which was designed to examine the connection of salt intake to high blood pressure, looked at 50 different populations spread across 30 countries and found that obesity was proportionately related to salt consumption. Subsequent studies investigating salt and blood pressure (DASH)[4] also found that with less salt in your food, body weight goes down. Also of note, tribes living in isolation, such as the Yanomami of the Amazon, that have never added salt to their food do not have the weight problem we are facing.

Some of the weight is related to salt and water retention. As we saw earlier in this book, excess salt consumed is balanced by retention of fluid. Weight gain during pregnancy happens for similar reasons. The baby may weigh only six pounds, but

3   Stamler J. The INTERSALT Study: Background, Methods, Findings and Implications. *The American Journal of Clinical Nutrition.* February 1997, Vol. 65 no. 2 626S–642S, http://ajcn.nutrition.org/content/65/2/626S.abstract.

4   Heller M. *The Dash Diet Weight Loss Solution: 2 Weeks to Drop Pounds, Boost Metabolism, and Get Healthy (A DASH Diet Book),* Grand Central Life & Style, 2012.

the mother gains as much as 20 pounds or more due in large measure to how much water she's retaining. This fluid retention and the related rise in blood pressure are big concerns during pregnancy and have potentially dangerous consequences if unchecked.

When you start cutting back on salt, the initial weight loss comes from losing the excess water in the body. Long-term weight reduction comes from eating less food. That's simple to understand. And that's exactly where the salt comes back in. You will eat a lot more of a salted rather than unsalted version of any food.

Test it yourself. Try eating unsalted peanuts or potato chips. After eating a certain amount of the unsalted version, you don't want any more. But salty chips or nuts? You cannot stop. The human brain puts up a stop sign to tell you when you have had enough. Salt makes you run through that stop sign, and you end up eating a lot more than you should. Unhealthy food choices, like junk food or fast food, make matters worse, since they're basically salt bombs.

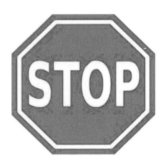

If you have any doubt about the role of salt in ready-made food, look how hard the salt and food-processing industries are fighting against any salt restriction. They're motivated only by one thing—profits—your health be damned.

In a 2002 report[5], Graham MacGregor and Hugh E. de Wardener argued that salt was being used by the food industry not because it was needed to preserve food, but because it was needed to make the taste of processed food tolerable. The authors of this report, which appeared in the *International Journal of Epidemiology*, make their case so strongly that I wanted you to be able to read at least part of it verbatim:

> Salt is no longer required for preservation. Unfortunately, with the development of processed foods, salt has once again become of great commercial importance, not only to the salt manufacturers and extractors, but also to the food and soft drinks industries. Many of the cheap processed foods are only palatable with the addition of large amounts of salt, the cheapest ingredient.
>
> It is not surprising, therefore, that commercial interests that represent the salt manufacturers and extractors, e.g. the Salt Institute in the US and the soft drinks industry, together with many sections of the food processing industry, have co-operated in perpetuating the idea that salt is not involved in hypertension.
>
> Nearly all government appointed bodies and nutrition experts who have considered the evidence have recommended a reduction in salt intake.

---

5   MacGregor, G., and de Wardener, H., "Commentary: Salt, Blood Pressure and Health," *International Journal of Epidemiology*, 2002, Vol. 31, Issue 2, pages 320–327.

When all of the evidence is considered from epidemiological, migration, intervention, treatment trials, genetic studies in humans and animal studies that relates salt intake to blood pressure and other harmful effects, the evidence is very strong. It is stronger than evidence for other dietary variables that are also important in cardiovascular disease, e.g. saturated fat intake and fruit and vegetable consumption.

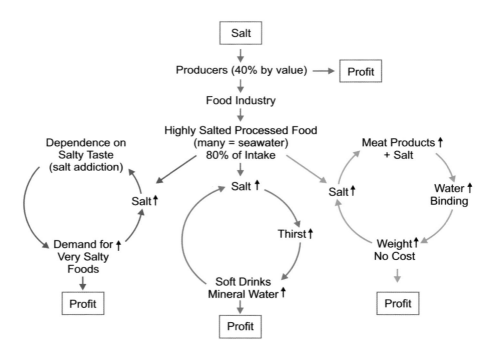

MacGregor, G., and de Wardener, H., "Commentary: Salt, Blood Pressure and Health," *International Journal of Epidemiology,* 2002, Vol. 31, Issue 2, pages 320–327. By permission of Oxford University Press.

In short, salt restriction can be a major factor in our battle against obesity and ensuing health problems. When you see the numerous weight-loss programs all over the media, you can tell most of them are just fads. Many of them are expensive and difficult to follow. We have learned from *Salt Kills* that reducing salt in your food is easy. It costs nothing and dramatically improves health while lowering your weight. Once you understand how harmful salt is and learn to enjoy the unadulterated taste of all that nature has to offer, you don't want to spoil the flavor of your food by adding salt. The Black American community has the most to gain from this simple measure and nothing to lose but weight.

Obesity Increases the Health Risks of the Following Conditions:

1. Coronary heart disease
2. Type 2 diabetes
3. Cancers (endometrial, breast and colon)
4. Hypertension (high blood pressure)
5. Dyslipidemia (for example, high total cholesterol or high levels of triglycerides)
6. Stroke
7. Liver and gallbladder disease
8. Sleep apnea and respiratory problems
9. Osteoarthritis (a degeneration of cartilage and its underlying bone within a joint)
10. Gynecological problems (abnormal menses, infertility)

Source: http://www.cdc.gov/obesity/adult/causes/index.html

By Disease, the Estimated Costs of Obesity-Related Illnesses:

Type 2 diabetes: $63.1 billion
Osteoarthritis: $17.2 billion
Coronary heart disease: $7.0 billion
Hypertension: $3.2 billion
Colon cancer: $2.8 billion
Post-menopausal breast cancer: $2.3 billion
Endometrial cancer: $790 million
Total cost: about $100 billion

Source: http://www.wvdhhr.org/bph/oehp/obesity/economic.htm

The saga continues. From gaining weight due to a salt habit, we move to losing calcium and the price Black America pays due to lost calcium.

Chapter

10

Osteoporosis

Black Americans, especially women, are just as likely as Caucasian Americans to develop osteoporosis. Despite the popular notion that they have thicker bones, fractures of bones due to osteoporosis are in fact commonly seen in the Black American community. For Black Americans, just like all Americans, once salt has been consumed, it punctures a hole in the kidneys, allowing calcium to escape. As a result, over time you inevitably end up with broken bones.

Black Americans, however, fare much worse than other ethnic groups when they break bones. After a hip fracture, for example, the overall mortality rate is already as high as 25 percent even with all of today's modern technology. Unfortunately, Black American women are twice as likely to die from consequences of a fractured hip. Let us do the math. That means that half of the Black American women who break a hip don't survive a seemingly simple bone fracture.

- Between 80 and 95 percent of fractures in Black American women over 64 are due to osteoporosis.
- Black American women are twice as likely as White American women to die following a hip fracture.
- Approximately 75 percent of Black Americans are lactose intolerant, which makes it difficult to consume enough bone-strengthening calcium.
- As Black American women age, their risk for hip fracture doubles approximately every seven years.
- Diseases more prevalent in the Black American population, such as sickle-cell anemia and systemic lupus, are linked to osteoporosis.
- Approximately 300,000 Black American women currently have osteoporosis.

Osteoporosis accounts for nearly all the fractures suffered by Black Americans once they are past 64 years of age. However, fractures are not the only damage that osteoporosis causes. Nerve damage—a common problem from collapsed bones like vertebrae—causes continuous, never-ending, severe pain. Think of what that must be like.

Certain diseases such as sickle-cell anemia and systemic lupus, which predominantly affect Black Americans, have been linked to the development of osteoporosis. Nearly 75 percent of Black Americans are also lactose intolerant, which makes getting enough calcium in the diet that much more difficult. And the kidneys lose that precious little bit of dietary calcium trying to get rid of the excess salt you keep adding to your food.

That's not a pretty picture, but the impact of eating salt-laden food, especially if you're a Black American, is not a pretty story.

Chapter

11

The Toll from the
Cradle to the Grave

By now, it should be amply clear that Black America pays a huge penalty for excess salt in food.

You may have come across the 2013 global brief on hypertension issued by the World Health Organization (WHO)[6]. The report, which was all over the news, says that there are at least one billion people in the world suffering from hypertension. The authors of the report focused on ways to solve this problem, which they call a "global crisis." What, then, about Black Americans? The word *crisis* doesn't begin to cover the horrible, multifaceted price Black Americans pay for disproportionately high blood pressure and all the complications that stem from that condition.

---

6   http://apps.who.int/iris/bitstream/10665/79059/1/WHO_DCO_ WHD_2013.2_eng.pdf.

Let's recap:

- High blood pressure, no matter how bad the consequences, is still only part of the damage that results from adding salt to food.
- Black American children suffer far more than most kids from acute asthmatic attacks. Just think about all those children gasping for breath.
- As they get older, young Black Americans in their most productive years of life run a higher risk of kidney failure and the prospect of living attached to a dialysis machine.
- Then comes the eventual, predictable and inevitable damage that high blood pressure does to the heart and brain. Heart attacks from blocked arteries, heart failure from an enlarged heart and strokes disproportionately disable untold numbers of Black Americans.
- In the later years, dementia and broken bones resulting from osteoporosis leave Black Americans severely disabled and dysfunctional at a much higher rate than they do Caucasian Americans.
- Along the way, Black Americans of all ages, especially women, are having to endure obesity-related health problems.

The case is clear. Salt is devastating the Black community. The toll of every single one of these salt-related health problems affects Black Americans several times more egregiously than it does Caucasian Americans. Every single one.

Chapter

12

A Tale of Opposites

Now let's talk about the toll that salt exacts in human terms. Meet Sarah (not her real name), an enterprising 37-year-old Black American professional who works in the high-tech industry. Her father's side of the family has always been quite healthy. At 83, her paternal grandmother still teaches Sunday school and even drives herself there and back—or anywhere else she wants to go, for that matter. All of her sisters—Sarah's paternal great-aunts—are still alive and most are equally active.

Sarah's maternal side of the family, however, is a completely different story. Her mother, now 63, was diagnosed with high blood pressure while still in her teens. Her blood pressure would often go up to or exceed 200/100 mm Hg. By the time she reached the age of 50 years, she had suffered multiple strokes, six of them in just one year.

Sarah's mom now has to contend with a handful of disabilities. She's also undergone a personality shift that has diminished her professional abilities. Although she used to run regional call centers for AT&T and had hundreds of people reporting to her, she's now overwhelmed by the idea of simply working part time as a receptionist. Other challenges include driving at night and negotiating heights due to vertigo (she won't visit her daughter because the house is 40 steps up from the sidewalk). But at least she's still alive. All but one of her six brothers are dead.

Sarah's five uncles all died young from multiple complications related to cardiovascular disease, heart failure and obesity caused and/or aggravated by salt. As a rule, they were very conscientious about taking care of themselves. They all had good jobs and most were quite successful. They tried to watch their diets. They went to exercise classes. They had consistent health care.

Neither they nor Sarah's mom fit the so-called typical picture of Black Americans in poor health. Like Sarah and her brother, they are (or were) well-educated, financially independent, in the upper income bracket. They've always had health care insurance coverage. Access to health care and visiting a physician have not been problems.

In short, this is not an economic issue. This is not an ignorance issue. This is not a compliance issue. This is, more than anything, a genetic issue turned deadly because of high-salt diets.

Where does Sarah fall in terms of her family history and salt sensitivity? She can't know, so she's not taking any chances. She remembers all too well those weekly visits to the convalescent home where her maternal grandmother and surviving great-uncle had been forced to move before Sarah was even born. Realizing that she does not know on which side of the family tree her health is going to fall, she watches her diet, choosing whole foods and avoiding salt, and is almost overly fixated on her fitness workouts. She is also largely the exception to the rule.

In our office, we see examples similar to Sarah's family. One segment of the population blames all of their heart problems on family history. While these people have a challenging family health history, like Sarah they should in fact be taking care of themselves more carefully by working hard to control all the known lifestyle risk factors. Foremost among those is simply avoiding salt. On the other hand, we have patients who say, "My grandfather lived to be 80." It is not easy to motivate this second category of people to follow healthy habits. They live with a false sense of security that they have surely inherited that same grandfather's genes.

This may explain the behavior of Sarah's brother, who is five years younger than she. Although he leads an active lifestyle, he smokes and refuses to believe that he needs to scrupulously watch his diet.

Sarah's mother, despite her history of strokes, is equally cavalier about her food choices. Although she doesn't think she eats badly, most of her meals come from a box or from a fast-food franchise, so they're loaded with salt, the very poison that has destroyed her health.

We know that salt intake predisposes Black Americans as a group to a host of diseases. Unfortunately, it is difficult to figure out who are the exceptions. While conducting research into salt sensitivity among rats at Brookhaven National Laboratory in Upton, New York, Dr. Dahl and his team studied more than 36,000 rats over the course of some 20 years. His experiments showed conclusively that some rats when fed a salty diet died very soon from complications related to high blood pressure. However, as we've previously discussed in this book, not all the rats were salt sensitive. Other rats, clearly on the opposite side of the spectrum, had no high blood pressure response to salt at all. These rats, which he called "salt resistant," went on to live an otherwise normal duration of life.

The extremely salt-sensitive rats developed a very high degree of high blood pressure and died within five months. The salt-resistant rats maintained blood pressure at normal levels and remained alive and well past 14 months. The outcomes in these rats clearly depended upon the degree of high blood pressure response to a salty diet. And only by gauging how quickly the rats died could Dr. Dahl determine a rat's salt sensitivity or resistance.

Dr. Dahl also concluded that human response to salt intake could also present with wide variation. Unfortunately, as with rats, the only way to determine your salt sensitivity or resistance is by seeing if you succumb to—or die from—conditions caused by salt. Are you willing to run that risk, especially in view of the fact that the vast majority of Black Americans are salt sensitive? For your sake, I sincerely hope not.

Chapter

13

The Trans-Atlantic Slave Trade and Salt Sensitivity

Salt sensitivity explains why salt exacts such a toll on the health of the Black American community. Salt sensitivity also explains why most Black Americans' high blood pressure responses to eating salt—along with myriad consequences suffered in response to salt intake—are so much more pronounced than other Americans'. But why are Black Americans so much more sensitive to salt than other populations?

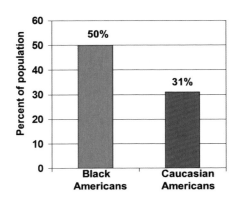

Salt Sensitivity

69

We know that the prevalence of high blood pressure and salt sensitivity is only about 15 percent among Black people living in Africa. That's much lower than the rates among descendents of former slaves now living in the U.S., the Caribbean and England. This finding has puzzled many researchers over the years. Clearly, something happened to those Africans who were forcibly removed from their home countries in chains. That something was a horrific journey called the Middle Passage.

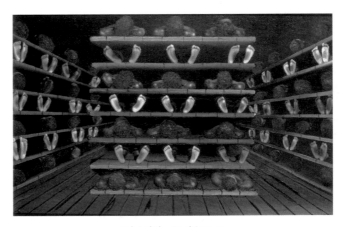

"Sheol" by Rod Brown

In the mid-19th century, about 13 million Africans were stolen from their homes and shipped from the west coast of Africa across the Atlantic to North America, England and the Caribbean. Sources say that at least 15 percent and possibly many more did not survive the trans-Atlantic voyage. Even more captives died shortly after reaching land.

Historians point out that dehydration was the main reason for these deaths. Not only did the slaves not have water to drink, they lost more water in perspiration due to being transported in

The Trans-Atlantic Slave Trade and Salt Sensitivity

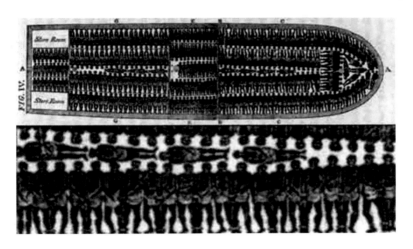

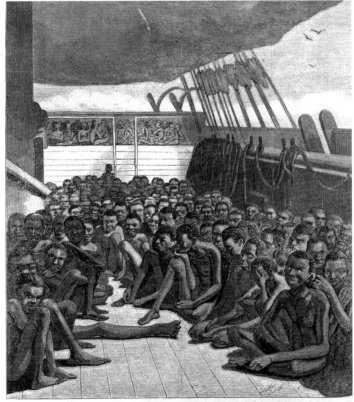

THE SLAVE DECK OF THE BARK "WILDFIRE," BROUGHT INTO KEY WEST ON APRIL 30, 1860.—[FROM A DAGUERREOTYPE.]

horrendously hot, humid conditions. Gastrointestinal diseases causing vomiting and dysentery were also common among slaves during the transport, causing further water loss. These catastrophic conditions are extensively documented.

African Blacks who had the ability to conserve salt (i.e., who were salt sensitive) had a better chance of surviving the ordeal. To balance the salt concentration in our body fluids, our bodies conserve extra water as well. Those of us who are salt sensitive do this more than others. In short, the surviving slaves' salt sensitivity likely saved them from the dehydration that killed so many others.

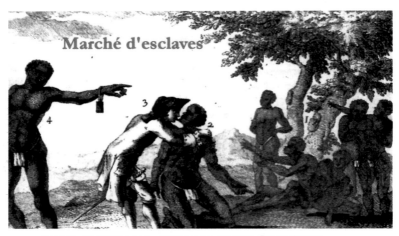

Slave trader licking a slave's face to assess his fitness for the voyage across the Atlantic. Source: Chambon, Le Commerce de l'Amérique par Marseille (Avignon, 1764).

Even in the 19th century, slavers realized that salt sensitivity among potential slaves to be transported was desirable. Just take a look at the picture of a slave trader licking the face of a captured African to determine how likely he would be to survive the inhumane conditions at sea.

While it is very likely that salt sensitivity proved to be a survival mechanism at one point in this shameful history, the same salt sensitivity has caused devastating health problems for Black Americans descended from slaves. It's worth noting that the children of newly arrived African immigrants have lower blood pressure than children who are descendants of slaves.

Dr. Dahl way back in the 1960s demonstrated that among rats salt sensitivity is heritable. Although a specific gene responsible for salt sensitivity has yet to be identified, it seems very reasonable to conclude that the slave trade and the Middle Passage have a lot to do with the present-day high blood pressure and its consequences among African Americans. This conclusion, however, does not sit well with everyone.

Chapter

14

The Controversy

Any talk of the slave trade, in whatever context, understandably touches a nerve. It is noteworthy that when the connection between salt-induced high blood pressure in salt-sensitive Black Americans and slavery was first mentioned on *The Oprah Winfrey Show*, it evoked many emotions.

The tone of some of the opposition to the salt sensitivity–slave trade connection can best be exemplified by a *Los Angeles Times* op-ed column on May 17, 2007, titled "Oprah's Unhealthy Mistake." In very caustic language, it essentially vilified Oprah for bringing up this salt sensitivity–slave trade connection, which, according to this piece, had long been debunked. The column, along with a few others, argued that this type of discussion unnecessarily diminishes the focus on socioeconomic disparities suffered by African Americans.

The author of the *Los Angeles Times* piece did not seem to take into account years of research done by Dr. Dahl and others at the Brookhaven National Laboratory on multiple subjects related to salt and high blood pressure. He also ignored another noteworthy report from Harvard University published in 2005. This report, titled "Racial Differences in Life Expectancy: The Impact of Salt, Slavery, and Selection,"[7] which was put together by a team of 24 professionals at Harvard University and features an extensive list of references, addresses in great depth the impact of the slave trade on present-day health care disparities. The report also specifically addresses the issue of salt sensitivity.

A better use of this space in the *Los Angeles Times* and other publications would have been to participate in educating their readership about high blood pressure. Taking a cue from Oprah's show, they could have helped Black Americans and everybody else to understand the dangers of salt consumption.

A 2013 report from Georgia Health Sciences University Institute of Public and Preventive Health[8] also deals with the relationship of salt sensitivity and high blood pressure among Black American test subjects from Atlanta. This report states that Black Americans of African descent can retain salt in response to stress, leading to high blood pressure. With a sin-

---

7   Further reading: Racial Differences in Life Expectancy: The Impact of Salt, Slavery, and Selection, David M. Cutler, Roland G. Fryer, Jr., and Edward L. Glaeser, Harvard University and NBER. March 1, 2005. isites.harvard.edu/fs/docs/icb.topic98848.files/salt_science_submission_3-01.pdf.

8   Harshfield GA, Hanevold C, Kapuku GK, Dong Y, Castles ME, Ludwig DA. The Association of Race and Sex to the Pressure Natriuresis Response to Stress. *Ethnicity & Disease*. Summer 2007;17(3):498–502.

gle stressful challenge, salt-sensitive Black Americans retain as much as 160 mg of sodium, which results in a rise in blood pressure of up to 7 mm Hg. Unlike test subjects of other ethnic origins whose blood pressure lowered when the source of stress was removed, the higher blood pressure sustained by salt-sensitive Black Americans did not return to the baseline.

Despite this devastation caused by salt sensitivity, Black Americans, the most affected group of people, do not generally seem to be aware of this problem. We need to do all we can to focus attention on preventing the deadly consequences of this salt sensitivity.

Chapter

15

Dos & Don'ts

By now, you should be convinced to stay away from adding any salt to your food. But if you have already been using salt for decades, some damage has already been done. So it is time to see the doctor. Here are a few tips for you to follow so that you can help your doctor help you.

1. **Check your blood pressure at home**: You must have heard of *white coat syndrome*. Blood pressure (BP) taken in the doctor's office can be higher than what your normal blood pressure really is. As a result, using the BP reading in the doctor's office to make adjustments in your medications is not a good idea. Nowadays you can get a home BP gizmo from any pharmacy. They are inexpensive, easy to use and quite reliable. Remember, the normal BP needs to be at or below 120/80. Once your BP crosses over

140/90, you have high blood pressure and you need medications. In between those numbers, you have pre-hypertension.

2. **Check your BP three times a day**: Your blood pressure range varies quite a bit during the course of the day. Making treatment decisions based on a single reading of BP in a day is not a good idea. If you have high blood pressure and are already on medications, you should check your BP three times a day: early morning, mid-afternoon and before bedtime. You must record these BP and heart rate readings for at least a week before your doctor's appointment. This information will help your doctor choose the correct medications for your high blood pressure.

3. **Check your weight every day**: This is a daily record of your eating habits. You know by now that salt will make you retain water. A morning change in weight will keep you honest. A sudden increase in weight may also be the earliest sign of heart failure and this will help you seek medical attention before a disaster happens.

4. **Engage with your medical team**: To provide information that can help improve interactions with your physician(s), especially for those of you with high blood pressure, I sought advice

from multiple primary care physicians. The physicians I regularly interact with are quite familiar with the special circumstances inherent in managing the blood pressure in Black Americans, since detecting and managing high blood pressure is job number one for physicians in America. Every time you go to a doctor, you get a blood pressure check even before you actually see the doctor. Regardless of ethnicity, the most common reason for pervasive undetected and undertreated high blood pressure is not seeing a physician. That's often not your fault. My primary care colleagues tell me that realistically no insurance company or the government will cover the frequency of doctor's office visits required to adequately manage high blood pressure.

Given the special circumstances of the unforgiving, raging high blood pressure among Black Americans, you can imagine the magnitude of this issue. Your best protection lies in your ability to engage with your medical team in a proactive way when you do get to see them.

- Be prepared for the doctor's office visit.
- Take records of your blood pressure, pulse rate and weight with you.
- Write down all the questions you have instead of simply trusting your memory.
- Gather as much information about your health as possible. Be aware that because

blood pressure in Black Americans is more aggressive and a different variety, it doesn't respond to the same medications used for Caucasian Americans. Consensus guidelines spell out which medications to use for Black Americans with high blood pressure.

- Take notes of the answers and the changes in medications.
- If possible, take a family member or a friend with you each time you see the doctor.
- Seek answers to your questions in a manner that reflects your own engagement with your health and not in a way that puts your caregiver in a defensive posture.
- Don't look for a pill for every health problem you have. Always ask, "What can I do instead of simply taking one more pill?"

5. **Heart failure clinics:** If you have been dealing with high blood pressure for a while, heart failure is definitely in your future. The most common reason for admission to a hospital for Americans over the age of 65 is heart failure. The most common reason for readmission is also heart failure. The hospitals and doctors often call heart failure patients "round-trippers"

because they return so frequently. One of the well-recognized reasons for persistent and recurrent heart failure happens to be inadequate after-discharge management of heart failure. In response, many health care systems are coming up with specialized "heart failure clinics." If you have this type of facility available to you, it is worth your consideration to keep your heart failure better monitored and better controlled. That can help keep you out of the hospital.

6. **Pre-hypertension—time to take action**: If your blood pressure is above normal but below the level where you would be placed on high blood pressure medications, you have "pre-hypertension." A BP reading below 140/90 mm Hg and above 120/80 mm Hg puts you in the category of pre-hypertension. This phase is the last chance you will get before you end up on a never-ending long road to high blood pressure medications and complications. One pill is just the beginning, and even that doesn't always work. Unfortunately, too many people don't even question this "solution." If I were to tell you that you needed a major surgery, you would consider the pros and cons, ask many questions, get second and third opinions and so on. But you probably wouldn't have the same degree of concern if the doctor told you that you needed a medication that you would have to take forever.

What a mistake! If you ever look up any of these medications, the long list of complications you will find in small print have actually happened to real individuals. It bears repeating: The very first time you are told that you need to be placed on pills, ask yourself: "What can I do so that I don't need to take these pills?" This is your golden opportunity to take a good look at your health habits and correct the problems before they go any further.

Rabindranath Tagore, a famous philosopher and Nobel Laureate from India, said it best: *Quinine will take care of malaria, but who will take care of quinine?*

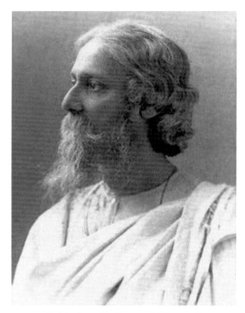

Rabindranath Tagore (1861–1941)
Nobel Prize in Literature, 1913

Conclusion

Many Black Americans are unaware of the problem of high blood pressure and its devastating effects. Despite the controversy, they are even less aware of the theorized relationship between salt sensitivity and the slave trade. This does not come as a surprise to me, as I talk with many African American health care providers and patients on a regular basis.

The big issue that has gotten lost is that Black Americans are indeed much more salt sensitive than Caucasian Americans. As a result, whether or not that salt sensitivity is the result of the trans-Atlantic slave trade survival mechanism, Black Americans suffer much higher rates of health problems from salt-induced high blood pressure. There is no controversy about that. It's the plain, sad truth.

Instead of engaging in a debate about the origins of salt sensitivity, Black Americans need to be informed about how salt is decimating their health in a way they can relate to. And the food-processing and beverage industries need to be forced to change.

Even after two centuries, overcoming many of the socio-economic barriers that hinder Black Americans continues to be a challenge. This book offers a simple and virtually free solution to at least one crushing problem. Prompting Black Americans to cut the salt in their diets could trigger a profound and lasting improvement in the health and well-being of under-served Black communities.

Won't you help?

In fact, we appeal to all influential people who care about the health of Black America to use their well-earned fame to promote this worthy cause. The knowledge about salt-induced high blood pressure and how that decimates the health of so many Black Americans has been around for several decades. Yet when I tell my medical colleagues or my Black American patients that they may have salt-induced high blood pressure, the answer, disappointingly is nearly always, "I did not know that." Therefore, a lot more needs to be done to spread the word. Can you imagine, empowered by this information, what would happen if Black Americans were to just cut the salt in their food? The state of Black America's health would improve dramatically with this single step.

Of course, reducing or eliminating salt consumption—especially when it comes to many Black Americans—isn't just a matter of putting down the salt shaker. Black Americans disproportionately consume large quantities of salt-laden processed foods, which are less expensive.

We've known for years that the majority of the excess salt we consume (80 percent) comes from processed foods. There is no legitimate excuse for adding so much salt in food processing. However, the food-processing industry, acting in the manner of the tobacco industry of yesteryear, shows little interest in cutting salt in processed food. For example, a 2013 study evaluating kids' meals available at fast-food chains determined that a mere 3 percent are healthy. That's up from 1 percent in 2006, but that's not much of an improvement, since 97 percent of fast-food meals designed for children still aren't at all good for them[9].

Many Black Americans live in neighborhoods that don't offer cheap, healthy choices. Why should inexpensive food equal salty and highly processed food? Why should it cost less to make processed food than fresh? And why is salt added to processed foods like bread, lunch meats and cheese in the first place? Don't tell me it's used for preservation. That is a poor excuse to cover up a profit motive. Studies have shown that salt causes people to eat more. People who eat more buy more. That, in large measure, explains the presence of so much salt in our pre-prepared food.

By simply educating the Black American community about the dangers of salt intake, we have the potential to dramatically impact the health of Black America—and indeed the health of the nation and the world.[10] It will be Black America that will rise and bring the food-processing industry to its knees. It will be Black America that will bring help to protect all food consumers by forcing meaningful legislation. It will be Black America that saves itself and the rest of the world.

9   http://cspinet.org/new/201303281.html.

10   Further reading: Racial Differences in Life Expectancy: The Impact of Salt, Slavery, and Selection, David M. Cutler, Roland G. Fryer, Jr., and Edward L. Glaeser, Harvard University and NBER. March 1, 2005. isites.harvard.edu/fs/docs/icb.topic98848.files/salt_science_submission_3-01.pdf.

For More Information

In this book, we've focused on how salt radically compromises the health of Black Americans. For more details about why consuming salt is so dangerous, please pick up a copy of my first book, *Salt Kills*. You'll find information about the book at saltkills.com.

Praise for *Salt Kills*

"Extremely well researched, unquestionably persuasive, and a great contribution to the health and well-being of the nation."
—Michael D. Connelly, president and CEO of Catholic Health Partners (CHP)
Michael D. Connelly, president and CEO of the nonprofit CHP, runs one of the largest health care systems in the country, overseeing some 100 different health care organizations across several states.

"I read Dr. Neravetla's book *Salt Kills* almost immediately after receiving it. It was very well set up and very well written. I read parts of this important contribution about the dangers of salt to my family as well."
—Dr. Robert Cerfolio, professor of surgery and chief of thoracic surgery, University of Alabama
Dr. Cerfolio, a well-recognized leader in thoracic surgery, has performed the highest volume of thoracic surgeries in the world four years running, performing more than 1,000 surgeries during each of those four years.

"Not to be missed. A splendid book. The proper response to Dr. Neravetla's book is to treat it as a prescription for more sensible shopping, cooking and eating—a message of global significance."

—Dr. J. Arthur Faber, professor of English, emeritus, Wittenberg University

About the Authors

Surender Reddy Neravetla, MD, FACS

Dr. Surender Neravetla, author of the critically acclaimed book *Salt Kills*, is the director of cardiac surgery at Springfield Regional Medical Center in Springfield, Ohio. While efforts by numerous organizations worldwide to create awareness about the dangers of adding salt to our food are yielding only limited success, Dr. Neravetla's book *Salt Kills*, along with his regular blog writings and frequent public presentations, has already encouraged thousands to reduce the salt in their food.

Dr. Neravetla obtained his medical degree from Osmania Medical College in Hyderabad, India. After arriving in the United States, he trained in general surgery at Jewish Hospital and Medical Center in Brooklyn, New York, and in cardiovascular surgery at the University of Cincinnati. In 1998, he started the heart surgery program at Springfield Regional Medical Center. The cardiac program has since been recognized nationally in the area of coronary artery bypass surgery for achieving the highest quality at the lowest cost.

Over the last three decades, Dr. Neravetla has performed more than 10,000 cardiac, vascular and lung surgeries. He is known for beating-heart bypass surgery, valve repairs and lung resections using state-of-the-art robotic technology. His vast expertise in carotid artery surgery makes him one of the country's most experienced surgeons in this area as well as one of the most successful when it comes to surgical results.

The Consumers' Research Council of America has recognized Dr. Neravetla as one of "America's Top Surgeons." His colleagues awarded him "The Golden Stethoscope," given to the hospital's most outstanding physician.

Despite Dr. Neravetla's surgical excellence, he is passionate about helping people avoid his services by improving their cardiovascular health.

Shantanu Reddy Neravetla, MD

Dr. Shantanu Neravetla graduated from the University of Louisville School of Medicine. He received a Bachelor of Science with high honors from Florida's University of Miami Honors Program. Over the years, Dr. Neravetla's research in various fields has resulted in numerous articles that have appeared in prominent peer-reviewed journals and conference publications. Dr. Neravetla's interest in preventive health dates back to his high school days when he campaigned as one of the nation's first American Red Cross Measles Initiative National Champions to raise awareness about measles and money for vaccinations around the world. In addition, Dr. Neravetla has gone on multiple international medical missions, including serving the indigent populations of the Amazon rainforest. In Ecuador, he noted drastic differences in blood pressure between rural and semi-urban populations. The University of Louisville honored Dr. Neravetla by presenting him with the Spirit of Service Award—he was the university's sole recipient.

Coming Soon

Cut salt from your diet and you've taken a huge step toward improving your health. What is next?

- What does eating right entail?
- Why has diabetes become increasingly common, even among vegetarians?
- What is the best way to get all the vitamins your body needs?
- What are antioxidants? How do they work?
- What does the disclaimer on the bottle of your favorite vitamin supplements really mean?
- What is the single most important thing we are doing wrong with our food, other than adding salt?
- What are the only kind of carbs we should be consuming?
- Is drinking tea good for you? What is the right way and what is the wrong way of making tea?
- Is milk good food? Is drinking it the best way to fight osteoporosis?
- How much protection from heart disease do cholesterol-lowering pills offer?
- And finally, what kind of exercise is most beneficial?

All this and more, illustrated and explained in our next book.